# YOUR KNOWLEDGE HAS VALUE

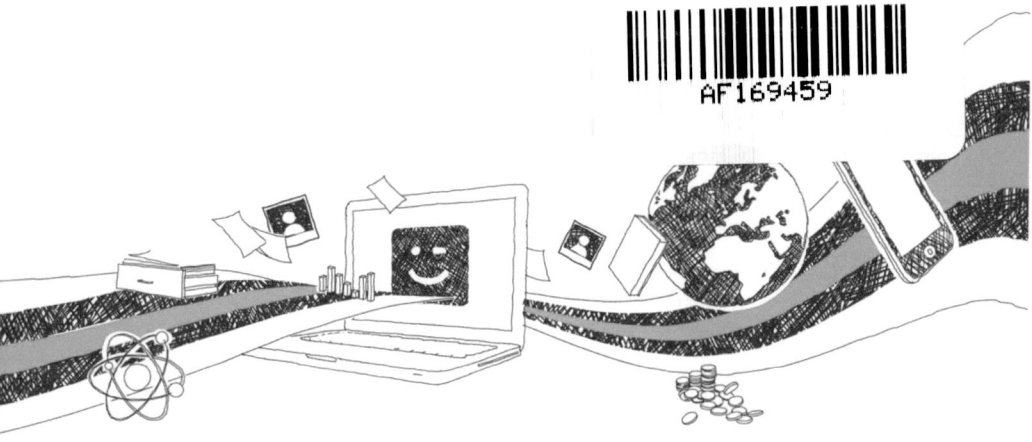

- We will publish your bachelor's and master's thesis, essays and papers

- Your own eBook and book - sold worldwide in all relevant shops

- Earn money with each sale

Upload your text at www.GRIN.com
and publish for free

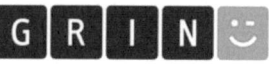

**Bibliographic information published by the German National Library:**

The German National Library lists this publication in the National Bibliography; detailed bibliographic data are available on the Internet at http://dnb.dnb.de .

This book is copyright material and must not be copied, reproduced, transferred, distributed, leased, licensed or publicly performed or used in any way except as specifically permitted in writing by the publishers, as allowed under the terms and conditions under which it was purchased or as strictly permitted by applicable copyright law. Any unauthorized distribution or use of this text may be a direct infringement of the author s and publisher s rights and those responsible may be liable in law accordingly.

**Imprint:**

Copyright © 2018 GRIN Verlag
Print and binding: Books on Demand GmbH, Norderstedt Germany
ISBN: 9783668736498

**This book at GRIN:**

https://www.grin.com/document/430705

Patrick Kimuyu

# Harmful Health Effects Associated with Aerial Spraying

GRIN Verlag

**GRIN - Your knowledge has value**

Since its foundation in 1998, GRIN has specialized in publishing academic texts by students, college teachers and other academics as e-book and printed book. The website www.grin.com is an ideal platform for presenting term papers, final papers, scientific essays, dissertations and specialist books.

**Visit us on the internet:**

http://www.grin.com/

http://www.facebook.com/grincom

http://www.twitter.com/grin_com

Harmful Health Effects Associated with Aerial Spraying

Name: Patrick Kimuyu

**Contents**

Introduction ............................................................................................................. 2

Literature Review .................................................................................................... 3

History of DDT ........................................................................................................ 4

Alternatives to Aerial Spraying ............................................................................... 6

Recommendations .................................................................................................. 7

Conclusion .............................................................................................................. 8

References ............................................................................................................ 10

Introduction

In the recent years, there has been a growing number of concerns about the cause and effect of using large scale pesticides for crop and general insect control. The concerns have also centered on how these pesticides are applied. There have been correlations made between aerial spraying and its impacts on the health of the general population. Notably, majority of pesticides used in the control of insects are not selective. For instance, Naled, Resmethrin and Malathion have been found to kill all insects. The numbers of insects killed include those help in keeping other insects under control. Additionally, aerial spraying threatens lives of aquatic animals and birds (Hester & Harrison, 2007). More importantly, agricultural production is under threat owing to increased usage of pesticides. This is because researchers argue that the continued usage of pesticides can lead to the development of resistance genes in organisms making them hard to control. As a result, farmers incur economic costs and decreased production.

With the growing concern over public health and safety, many ways we use to operate have either been changed or eliminated altogether. As examples, the use of lead in house paint and asbestos as an insulation product, have been eliminated. Their removal is highly controlled and regulated. Regulations have been developed to govern the installation of electrical circuits and plumbing product. These have been implemented because of the growing awareness over health and safety (Hester & Harrison, 2007).

Research has also found that some pesticides used in mosquitoes contribute to immune suppression. Ideally, the suppression of the human system can lead to allergies, cancers, autoimmune disorder and lupus. For instance, Malathion is the mostly used pesticide and can cause neurotoxicity. Malathion can also cause headaches, diarrhea and nausea (Hester & Harrison, 2007).

It is time to stop aerial spraying and find other, less damaging mechanisms to deal with insect infestations. There is a reason for using aerial spraying of fire retardants for forest fires. The result being everything under the airplane is covered, not just the fire. I am proposing that we should stop the usage of aerial spraying and adopt safer practices to control insects. Aerial spraying has serious ramifications to the population, and to the planet.

Literature Review

According to Oregon State University, farmers use about 77% of all pesticides in the US. 10% of pesticides are used annually on forests and lawns for bug control. Home gardeners are often some of the most extravagant users. The average US homeowner uses 2 - 6 times more pesticide per acre than do farmers (Patricia, 2012). The total amount of pesticides applied on farms in the US has increased 170% between 1964 and 1982. This is despite the amount of farmland decreasing. Continued usage of pesticides has lead to various problems. For instance, officials from Lyon County, Iowa most recently blame aerial spraying for the fish kill in an unnamed stream that flows into Otter Creek. Three aerial applicators were seen flying in the area the day of the fish kill (Iowa Department of Natural Resource, 2014). This is occurring all over the United States. People may turn a blind eye to it, think that it is a shame and move on with their lives. These fish kills are not only killing fish, they are other forms of wildlife that live and feed off the ecosystem in the area. More importantly, fish are the source of food and live hood to some communities. Reduction of the fish community owing to aerial sprays will affect such communities and hence the likelihood of conflicts. Further, failing to control the amount of pesticides entering lakes, oceans and rivers will reduce the oxygen levels needed in aerating water. Low level of aeration in drinking water can compromise the quality. Application of Pesticides in farm nears water masses can kill aquatic plants essential for the survival of fish and marine insects (Iowa Department of Natural Resource, 2014). As a result, marine animals can be forced to migrate to other places looking for food and end up exposing themselves to predators (Patricia, 2012).

An editorial entitled "The Dangers of Pesticides, Go Organic Instead", author Judith (2010) paints a grim picture of her personal experience with pesticides. The author grew up outside of Phoenix, Arizona. She recalls sitting outside with her family while crop dusters flew overhead. Her sister has been plagued with asthma and cancer. Both of her parents have battled cancer and her father died because of cancer. Judith (2010) herself has been suffering from immune problems and fibromyalgia. It is not certain that the pesticides were totally to blame. The fact the pesticides were applied by blanketing everything from the air certainly needs to be investigated. The results need to be forwarded to the legislative body so the appropriate actions will result (Judith, 2010). Why put something on our food that could lead to permanent health issues or even death? Judith (2010) points out that when the scientists went back to examine the atomic bomb testing sites in New York and New Mexico, they learned that every life form was killed. Plants and animals died, but the one living species that survived the atom bomb radiation were the insects. This is something to think about (Judith, 2010). Even though they are not using atomic bombs to kill off insects, can you imagine what chemicals are in the pesticides, and herbicides used to kill both plant and animals alike?

Judith (2010) states that the organic farmer knows they will lose a small portion of their crops to nature. Rabbits will attack your garden; potato beetles will eat some of your crop. Organic fruits and vegetables will not look as good as some that have been treated by chemicals. At what price are we willing to sacrifice so that our fruits and vegetables will look aesthetically pleasing? Reducing aerial sprays and encouraging organic farming will help in reducing the harmful effects of chemicals while at the same time safeguarding the environment.

### History of DDT

Dichlorodiphenyltrichloroethane (DDT) was discovered in a lab in 1873. It was not transformed into a pesticide until 1939. Dr. Paul Muller even won a Nobel Prize for this discovery. It was excessively used during WWII as a pesticide. After WWII, it was used on farms for insect control. Initially, DDT was an excellent product that transformed the agricultural sector. DDT aided in controlling insects seen to affect agricultural sectors. Some researchers argue that DDT is still an excellent product in controlling insects such as mosquitoes. This is because the product is cheap and highly effective in controlling malaria. It has also a long half-life and a broad spectrum of activity. However, DDT has been linked liver damage, reproductive complications and problems with the nervous problems (Duke University, 2010).

It was finally banned in 1972. Despite being banned 42 years ago, DDT is still used in other countries. Currently, the Great Lakes Region of America is seeing atmospheric deposition due to DDT use in other parts of the world. As DDT breaks down, it takes on other forms which are equally toxic, such as DDE and DDD. It takes 15 years for DDT to entirely break down in our environment. DDT also affects American's because it is used on the food that we import. It has also been found in fish that is imported into America. Infants can be exposed to DDT through their mother's breast milk (DDT, 2011).

*Harmful Effects of DDT*

The first effect of DDT usage is that it causes air and soil pollution. DDT drifty occurs when molecules suspended in the air are carried by wind to other areas leading to contamination. The volatility nature of the DDT increases chances of being blown away by wind into far places threatening wildlife. These threats increase during times of high temperatures and low humidity. The threat posed by DDT sprays has led to legislations, which require non-crop plants to serve as windbreaks. It is also vital to note that DDT usage can fumigate the soil resulting to the production of volatile organic compounds. These compounds react with other soil chemicals forming tropospheric ozone (Acton, 2012). The current research reveals that the usage DDT and other aerial sprays hinder nitrogen fixation in soil affecting the health of plants. Specifically, DDT interferes with legume-rhizobium chemical signaling reducing the plant yield. Essentially, root nodule formation reducing the usage of nitrogen fertilizers in the agricultural sector.

The second effect of DDT is that it poses a threat to the life of predatory birds and marine life. This is due to the lipophilic property of the chemical. DDT has the ability to be transferred in the food chain with apex predators standing a chance of accumulating more chemicals compared to other animals in the same habitat. The Centre for Disease Control detected DDT in almost all samples of human blood in the year 2005 raising fears among the public about the long-term impacts of chemical to their lives.

The usage of DDT will likely affect the marine life of many organisms. This is because DDT causes eggshell thinning and the potentiality of egg breakages and deaths. Evidently, the detection of DDT in egg shell is considered scientists as the core reason of declining populations of bald eagle, osprey, brown pelican and peregrine falcon (Patricia, 2012).

**Alternatives to Aerial Spraying**

With all of the bad side effects that we see with DDT, the time is now to take swift action to curb all of its uses. We are an intelligent species that needs to learn from our mistakes. By continuing using DDT, more people will suffer from its poisons. We have over one hundred years of evidence that proves DDT is a harmful substance (Tjeerdema, 2012). It seems backwards to combat insects that kill our crops with something that will kill us.

According to California Alliance to Stop the Spray, The California Department of Food and Agriculture ordered a massive aerial spray in 2007 in the San Francisco Bay region in an effort to control the Light Brown Apple Moth. The aerial spraying covered two counties that resulted in 600 people having a medical reaction to the spray. Within hours of the spraying 650 sea birds washed up dead on Monterey Bay. The aerial spraying was not to occur after a rain shower, yet it rained a few hours after the spraying. The Santa Cruz County experienced the largest red tide since the 1960's. There were large deposits of yellow foam on the seashores immediately following the aerial spraying in Santa Cruz County (Duke University, 2010). A large number of cats and rabbits died. Untold number of pollinators and bees were found dead.

Erecting wind turbines can help in developing a greener planet. This can be done by soliciting finances by companies such as Optimum Renewable from Des Moines, Iowa. The establishment of wind turbines will reduce emissions by 10% or more in California, Idaho, Colorado, Iowa, Kansa, Oregon, South Dakota, Vermont, Nebraska, Washington and Minnesota (AWEA, 2013).

Handpicking can help reduce the need to use pesticides. Basil and lavender are natural plants that repel mosquitoes and other flying insects. Additionally, there are beneficial insects and predators that can replace pesticides. Swallows eat moths, beetles and grasshoppers. Sparrows eat caterpillars and beetles. The robins enjoy eating grasshoppers. Encouraging these birds to live in and near the fields can cut the number of insects (Hond, Groenewegen & Straalen, 2008). Thus, it is vital that the US devotes times and resources to develop policies and laws capable of regulating the usage of aerial sprays.

Recommendations

It is the time we also take a leading role in abolishing the use of pesticides, herbicides, and the use of aerial, blanket application. I know that we are a nation that is on a path that will lead us into a greener environment. The use of toxic pesticides and the means by which they are applied has caught up with us. There does not need to be another fish kill, or persons suffering, to determine that the time to say good bye to pesticides and the use of blanketing aerial spraying is overdue. This is our home, and our responsibility.

This proposal can be implemented by embracing various measures. Firstly, I propose that the US makes use of biological control measures of insects. In this case, integrated pest management (IPM) programs should be implemented to help in reducing the usage pesticides. In addition, it is vital to adopt biological pest control strategies such as augmentation, conservation and importation. Currently, the importation of pest natural enemies stand at 40% and should be increased to bigger percentages. However, the government should reduce legal procedures required in importations of such pests. The usage of biological control measures will help in eliminating populations of agriculturally and ecologically invasive species (Horne & Page, 2008).

Secondly, strengthening agencies like the EPA and the Department of Pesticide Regulations will help in compelling manufacturers in availing components used in their products open for the public scrutiny will aid in implementing this proposal. Mostly, incomplete lists of substances to be sprayed become available to the public by Public Records Requests or accidental publications. The unelected bureaucrats do not want the exact spray mixtures to be open to public scrutiny. Unfortunately, the public is not allowed to know all of the ingredients, mixtures, and quantities that are to be sprayed on them because of trade secret laws. In the case of the 2007 LBAM spraying project, a list of ingredients for the biochemical pesticide was published in the September 28, 2007 edition of The Santa Cruz Sentinel newspaper. Because of that published article, the list of ingredients was available to the public for 14 days with no opposition from Suterra, the manufacturer of the biochemical pesticide. But when a judge in Monterey

County temporarily delayed the spray project due to the questionable health effects of one of the reported ingredients, Suterra immediately issued cession and desisted requests and demanded that all websites and all newspapers remove the list of ingredients from the public domain, claiming violations of trade secret laws. As demonstrated in this case and many others, manufacturer's rights to spray secret biochemical on urban and residential areas outweigh the public's right to safety and the public. Consumers have the 'Right to know'. When the laws are many to protect corporations but few to protect the individual, it is sometimes called corporate personhood. As a result, it is vital to strengthen the EPA in order to act against those manufactures' unwilling to offer information concerning the product to the public. The public has the authority to be educated about the composition of the product and the potential side effects. Manufactures' are supposed to be restricted from releasing the products in the market until they meet the required regulations. As a result, any side effects coming from their product will enable the government to compel such manufactures to offer compensation to the affected people.

Thirdly, the Title 50 Chapter 32 Sec. 1520A should be revised to allow for more experimentation on humans or the unwitting public. The federal government of the United States allows public and private sectors to conduct experiments on the people of this nation. To do so legally, all an agency must do is get congressional approval, as in a rider to legislation, and get permission from a local authority (the local dog catcher would meet the necessary requirements). Experiments are not usually disclosed to the public. The military claims secrecy under national security and corporations claim secrecy under trade secrets laws. A brief overview of recent human experimentations conducted on US residents (Hond, Groenewegen & Straalen, 2008).

Conclusion

In conclusion, it is vital to stop the usage of aerial spraying and develop safer practices to control insects. Evidently, aerial sprays cause far reaching consequences to the life of human being, wildlife, aquatic animals and plants. For instance, Officials from Lyon County have found that aerial sprays kill fishes and other marine animals. This can complicate the transfer of energy in food chain and quality of drinking water. Additionally, aerial spraying has been found to affect the health of human beings resulting to cancers, asthma and immune-related disorders. DDT remains the highly used aerial spray in the world. It was banned in 1972 in the US. However, the product continued being used in the agricultural production. From the issues discussed in this paper, I strongly believe that creating policies that encourage the usage of biological pest control methods instead of aerial sprays can lead to a stable ecosystem. Biological control of pest can be propped by implementing integrated pest control programs and physical methods.

**References**

Acton, Q. (2012). *Pesticides—Advances in Research and Application (2012 Edn)*. Atlanta, GA: Scholarly Editions.

American Wind Energy Association. (2013). *AWEA fact sheets: quick guides to wind energy. AWEA fact sheets: quick guides to wind energy.* Retrieved from http://awea.rd.net/Resources/Content.aspx?ItemNumber=873&navItemNumber=588

DDT. (2011). *EPA. Environmental Protection Agency.* Retrieved from http://www.epa.gov/pbt/pubs/ddt.htm

Duke University. (2010). *An Introduction. DDT: An Introduction.* Retrieved from http://people.chem.duke.edu/~jds/cruis_chem/pest/pest1.html

Hester, R., & Harrison, R. (2007). *Biodiversity under Threat.* London: Royal Society of Chemistry.

Hond, F., Groenewegen, P., & Straalen, N. (2008). *Pesticides: Problems, Improvements, Alternatives.* Hoboken, NJ: John Wiley & Sons.

Horne, P., & Page, J. (2008). *Integrated Pest Management for Crops and Pastures.* Oxford Street: Landlinks Press.

Iowa Department of Natural Resource. (2014). 2nd Lyon County fish kill thought to be caused by aerial spraying. *Sioux City Journal, 20*(2).

Judith, R. (2010). *The Dangers of Pesticide Exposure - Go Organic Instead. Hub Pages.* Retrieved from http://judithrizzo.hubpages.com/hub/The-Dangers-of-Pesticide-Exposure-Go-Organic-Instead

Patricia, M. (2012). *History of Pesticide. Oregon State University. Oregon State University.* Retrieved from http://people.oregonstate.edu/~muirp/pes

Tjeerdema, R. (2012*). Aquatic Life Water Quality Criteria for Selected Pesticides.* London, UK: Springer Science & Business Media.

# YOUR KNOWLEDGE HAS VALUE

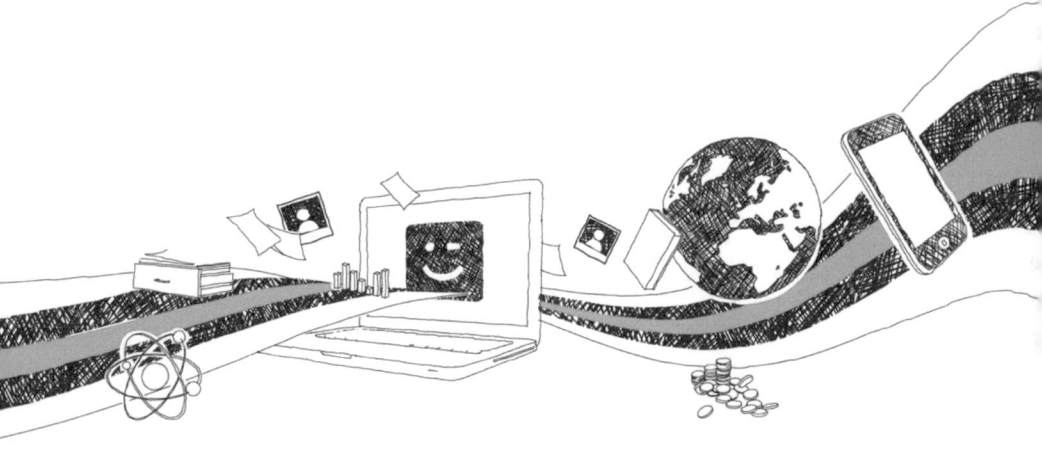

- We will publish your bachelor's and
  master's thesis, essays and papers

- Your own eBook and book -
  sold worldwide in all relevant shops

- Earn money with each sale

Upload your text at www.GRIN.com
and publish for free

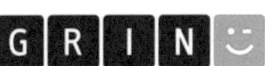